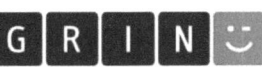

Therapeutic Benefits of Using Miswak

Nageen Akhtar

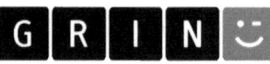

Bibliographic information published by the German National Library:

The German National Library lists this publication in the National Bibliography; detailed bibliographic data are available on the Internet at http://dnb.dnb.de.

ISBN: 9783389036242
This book is also available as an ebook.

Print and binding: Books on Demand GmbH, Norderstedt, Germany
Printed on acid-free paper from responsible sources.

The present work has been carefully prepared. Nevertheless, authors and publishers do not incur liability for the correctness of information, notes, links and advice as well as any printing errors.

GRIN web shop: https://www.grin.com/document/1478457

LITERATURE REVIEW ON MISWAAK

DR.NAGEEN AKHTAR

ABSTRACT

Miswaak has been considered a wonder stick from ancient times because of its immense benefits.Following is a review article considering numerous aspects on miswaak including:

❖ Biological components of miswaak(salvadora persica)and their effects on oral health.
❖ Studies showing comparison between miswaak and toothbrush use.
❖ Epidemiological surveys(effects on different oral health care parameters including caries, plaque and gingival scoring indices,pain and saliva secretion).
❖ Comparison of fresh and old miswaak effects on oral health and index scores
❖ Comparison between different types of miswaak and differences in their effects, chemical composition and anti microbial activity.

BIOACTIVE COMPONENTS OF MISWAAK(*SALVADORA PERSICA*)AND THEIR EFFECTS ON ORAL HEALTH

Miswaak biological components:

Chemical analysis of various components of miswak (*Salvadora persica*)

Chemical substance	Reference
B-sitosterol and m-anisic acid	[22]
Chlorides, salvadora and gypsum; organic compounds, such as pyrrolidine, pyrrole, and piperidine derivatives	[23]
Flavonoids, including kaempferol, quercetin, quercetin rutin, and a quercetin glucoside	[24]
Glycosides, such as salvadoside and salvadoraside	[25]
Sodium bicarbonate	[26]
Resin large amounts of salts containing chlorine	[27]
Trimethylamine, an alkaloid, chlorides, high amounts of fluoride, silica, sulfur, Vitamin C	[28]

Beneficial role of various chemicals present in miswak (*Salvadora persica*)

Chemical substance	Mode of action	Beneficial role	Reference
Fluoride	Antimicrobial	Prevent caries	[29,30]
Vitamin C	Healing/repair	Healing of oral tissues	[27,31]
Silica	Abrasive	Removes stains and plaque	[27,32]
Tannic acid	Antifungal	Reduces *Candida albican*	[32,33]
Sulphur	Bactericidal	Reduces bacterial count	[34,35]
Sodium bicarbonate	Abrasive	Used as dentifrice	[30,36]
Calcium	Inhibits demineralization and promotes remineralization	Buffering role in the oral cavity	[30,33]
Alkaloid (salvadorine)	Bactericidal	Stimulatory effect on gingiva	[28]
Essential oils	Antiseptic	Disinfects the oral cavity	[27,34]
Benzylisothiocynate	Preventive agent	Prevents against genotoxic and carcinogenic compounds	[30,37]
Resins	Forms a layer on enamel surface	Makes teeth resistant to caries attack	[32]
Chloride	prevents calculus deposition on teeth surfaces; inhibits demineralization and promotes remineralization	Buffering role and maintains favorable pH of the oral cavity	[27,31]

- Use of miswak is also found to regulate peristaltic movements, lowers high-density lipoprotein cholesterol and improves appetite.(1)

Table 2: Chemical components of Miswak

Chemical properties	Oral health benefits/effects
Fluoride	Remineralization of tooth structure from the repeated use of Miswak, which releases containing sap
Silica	An abrasive material to remove tooth stain
Tannins	A phenolic compound that has an astringent effect and premolar saliva production
Resins	Amorphous products that form a protective layer over the enamel to prevent caries
Alkaloids	Nitrogenous organic compounds found in plants, which have a bactericidal effects and stimulatory actions on the gingival, e.g., Salvodorine
Essential oils	Benzyl nitrite, eugenol, thymol, isothymol, eucalyptoi, isoterpinolene and g-caryophyllene that have anti bacterial effects; characteristic aroma; carminative action, mild bitter taste stimulates the flow of saliva
Sulphur compounds	Compounds have a pungent taste and smell and bactericidal effect
Vitamin C	Ascorbic acid promotes healing and tissue repair
Sodium bicarbonate	A compound used as a dentifrice, because of its mild abrasive properties
Calcium	A mineral that inhibit enamel demineralization and promotes remineralization
Chloride	An element that inhibit calculus formation and helps in removing extrinsic tooth stains
Benzyl isothiocyanate	A chemotherapeutic agent with anti-carcinogenic properties

(2)

- Miswak contains many chemical components which can be activated while in the mouth by saliva, for instance, **Cl-** leaching into saliva from miswak may mediate the innate host defense systems in human saliva. Cl-, I- and SCN- (pseudohalides) are substrates for salivary peroxidise and/or the myeloperoxidase hydrogen peroxide antimicrobial system. The peroxidase-hydrogen-peroxide-chloride system is a part of the innate host defense that is mediated by polymorphonuclear leukocytes in humans. It has been shown that the latter system was more bactericidal against *Aggregatibacter actinomycetemcomitans* than with the myeloperoxidase-thiocyanate and hydrogen peroxide system. Recently, it has been indicated that the oxidation product of lactoperoxidase and myloperoxidase with I- and/or Cl- was bactericidal against *Porphyromonas gingivalis, Fusobacterium nucleatum* and *Streptococcus mutans* .The lower levels of *Prevotella intermedia* and *Fusobacterium nucleatum* in the miswak users may be attributed to its Cl- and SCN- content.(3)

- **Salvadorins and alkaloids** have antimicrobial and mild stimulating effects on gums. The toothbrush plant can prevent diseases caused by periodontal bacterial pathogens due to inhibitory activities on proteases and peptidases enzymes.

- **Trimethylamine** prevents the accumulation of food particles between the teeth. **Methylamine** as an abstergent improves mouth ulcers, makes healthy growth, and causes modifying and reducing the index of hydrogen ion activity in the oral cavity that indirectly affects the oral microbial growth.

- There are significant amounts of **sodium chloride and potassium chloride** along with sulfur in the persica plant. These substances, in addition to mild disinfecting role, cover the enamel through adhesion properties, prevent tooth decay and dental germ, and help to remove stains and deposits on the tooth surface.

- There is **sulfur** at a concentration of 4.73% in the ash resulting from the plant roots, which alone has a bactericidal effect.

- **Fluoride** strengthens the tooth enamel structure. Some studies have reported that the plant root soaking in water causes release of fluoride at concentrations between 0.07 and 0.1 µg/ml.

- **Tannins** in persica plant have strengthening property for the gums, and help to reduce gingivitis. Flavonoids and tannins, in addition to having strong anti-ulcer effect for gums, inhibit the activity of glucosyltransferase to prevent the formation of calculus and gingivitis.

- **Vitamin C and sitosterol** have potential role in boosting blood flow to the capillaries of the gums, restoration, healing and preventing the gingivitis. Investigations also indicated that frequent chewing persica plant root causes the release of fresh resins with anti-cancer effects. The resin also protects the teeth against dental diseases by creating a coating layer.

- **Silica** plays an important role in teeth whitening, and vitamin C is widely used in controlling oral infection. Based on studies carried out in some countries, anti-microbial and anti-plaque effects of wood powder prepared from Arak were the same best form of commercial toothpastes. In recent years, many pharmaceutical manufacturers produced toothpastes and mouthwash drops containing extracts of roots and trunks of the Arak tree.

- Calcium saturation, especially **calcium bicarbonate**, in the saliva caused by chewing the wood of persica plant roots allows faster regeneration of tooth enamel.
- Some studies have reported that high concentrations of **sulfate** in the toothbrush plant extract prevent the growth of *Candida albicans*.

- **Thiocyanate compounds** in the plant has a strong influence on salivary peroxidase system with antimicrobial effect and gives rise to specific and nonspecific tissue resistance mechanisms against infections.

- The main anti microbial component of miswaak according to a study was found to be Benzyl isothiocyanate(4).
- Extraction of **benzylisothiocyanate (BITC)** from persica plant root suggests that BITC is a final anti-cancer and anti-genotoxic product resulting from the enzymatic hydrolysis of glucosinolate contained in the persica plant.(5)

- Upon the plant tissue damage,BITC is released as an effector molecule of the plant defence system through hydrolysis of benzyl glucosinolate by the enzyme myrosinase.The plant enzyme myrosinase and its substrates glucosinolates are are physically separated in plants.So,plant tissue damage is a pre requisite for releasing isothiocyanates.The cruciferous vegetables of the genera Brassica and Sinapis are rich in benzyl glucosinolates.Hence,BITC is released into the oral cavity and gastrointestinal tract upon consumption of uncooked cruciferous vegetables.The same mechanism appears active in the release of BITC when a miswaak stick is chewed on prior to mechanical cleansing of the teeth. As boiled miswaak sticks lose antibacterial activity,most likely due to inactivation of the myrosinase,this assumption is confirmed.(4)
- The BITC is an inhibitory chemical substance, and its presence at the site is thought to be effective in preventing reach to the target tissue or response to carcinogens. The concentration of 133.3 µg/ml of BITC is virucide and manages to destroy herpes simplex virus 1 and a large range of bacteria, as well as it can prevent the growth and acid production by *Streptococcus mutans*. Investigations have demonstrated that antibacterial activity of toothbrush plant is selective and ideal, especially on anaerobic microorganisms such as *S. mutans* that causes tooth decay, and even fungi such as candida as well as can eliminate 97% of mouth germs in a short time.

- This active ingredient of toothbrush stick called **benzyl isothiocyanate** dissolves in saliva after entering the mouth; this substance combines with one atom of oxygen in H2O2 produced by oral microbial activities and finally produces water and the new composition of benzyl isothiocyanate oxide. As a result, hydrogen peroxide in the saliva neutralizes, reducing damage to the tissues of the oral mucosa. The produced benzyl isothiocyanate oxide has stronger antimicrobial effect than benzyl isothiocyanate. The benzyl isothiocyanate is secreted naturally in small amounts by the salivary glands in the mouth, and this is one of the wonders of the toothbrush plant that is unique.

- Among the compounds of Arak, **anisic acid** helps for chest sputum removal.

- In addition, there are some **ascorbic acid and sitosterol**, which strengthen blood vessels leading to gingivitis.

- Also, 1% **aromatic oil** can be found in this plant that leads to fragrant mouth.

- Another substance is **enterolithon** that is useful in strengthening appetite, eating and in regulating bowel movement.

- Al Lafi (1995) reported that the persica plant derivatives have strong germicidal effects, particularly Streptococcus and *Staphylococcus aureus*.

- Almas and his colleagues also found that *Enterococcus faecalis* decreased in the mouths of subjects who had used the toothbrush plant about a month compared with those who had used shortly.

- Albaghie compared the bactericidal properties of aqueous and alcoholic extracts of toothbrush plant roots and concluded that ethanol extract was strong bactericide than aqueous extract.The persica plant in addition to maintaining and improving oral and dental health helps to digest food; for example, a rather bitter taste of oils in the plant triggers and secretes more saliva, resulting in better activities of other digestive enzymes.The toothbrush plant contains a large amount of sharp-taste substance, which is antiseptic, abstergent, inhibitors of bleeding gums and gum reinforcing.(5)

- Calcium saturation in saliva inhibits demineralization and promotes remineralisation of tooth enamel.High chloride content reduces calculus formation and activates amylase to limit caries formation. (6)

- *S. persica* as a root canal irrigant has better antimicrobial properties when compared to chlorhexidine gluconate and sodium hypochlorite. Recent studies and evidences have suggested that *S. persica* has good antimicrobial activity with a low level of cytotoxicity and causing no significant damage to the host cells at an optimal therapeutic concentration.*S. persica* (15%) exhibited an effective antimicrobial activity against aerobic and an-aerobic organisms. Further, a recent study by Almas compared cytotoxicity of chlorhexidine gluconate and miswak extracts on mouse fibroblasts. The miswak extracts was less cytotoxic and cells viability with miswak extracts was greater than chlorhexidine gluconate.These evidences altogether supported the idea of using miswak extracts as an endodontic irrigation solution. The incidence of caries is notably low in miswak users owing to the presence of a strong antimicrobial thiocyanate agent, accompanied by other chemicals such as sodium chloride, potassium chloride, saponin, tanins. The extracts of miswak showed significant reduction in the growth of cariogenic bacteria.The miswak soaked in 0.1–0.5% NaF solutions help to reduce the cariogenic bacterial count and dental decay. Fluoride is well known for antimicrobial activates in the oral cavity.

- A study by Mohamed and Khan concluded that antioxidant enzymes in miswak **(catalase, peroxidase, polyphenols oxidase)** attribute to antioxidant property of *S. persica*. Thus, synergistic effect of antioxidant compounds and enzymes makes miswak a good oral hygiene maintaining tool. Another study by Ibrahim *et al.* showed that antioxidant property, content of flavonoid and phenolic was more in miswak from southern region compared to the central region of Saudi Arabia.

Gupta *et al.* performed antioxidant and phytochemical study on *S. persica* and reported that the chloroform extract from miswak showed most antioxidant effect *in vitro* followed by ethanolic extract.(1)

- Al Lafi and Ababneh tested the antibacterial activity of *Salvadora persica* against some oral aerobic and anaerobic bacteria and reported that the extract of these sticks had a drastic effect on the growth of *Staphylococcus aureus,* and a variable effect on other bacterial species.(6)

- According to a study strong anti bacterial effects of miswaak were tested against oral microorganisms associated with periodontitis and caries and it was found that the miswak exhibited stronger antibacterial activity against the Gram-negative bacteria tested in this study than the Gram-positive bacteria evaluated, as evidenced by the pronounced differences in inhibition zones associated with the Gram-negative species A.actinomycetemcomitans, P. gingivalis, H. influenzae, and the Gram-positive species S. mutans and L. acidophilus.(7)

- According to the results of a study both fresh miswaak and essential oil miswaak extract had a strong anti bacterial activity against gram negative bacteria including some oral pathogens such as Porphyromonas gingivalis Aggregatibacter actinimycetemcomitans.(4)

STUDIES SHOWING COMPARISON BETWEEN MISWAAK AND TOOTH BRUSH/TOOTH PASTE:

Salient difference between miswak and toothbrush

	Miswak	Toothbrush
Source	Natural	Synthetic
Dentifrice needed	No	Yes
Cost[2]	Cheap	Can be expensive (for public)
Efficiency[20,69]	Good	Good
Gingival recession	No if correct technique is used[70,71]	Yes[72]
Tooth abrasion[70,73]	No if correct technique is used	Yes
Disinfection needed	No (as it has disinfectant property itself)[69]	Yes[71,74]
Saliva stimulation	Yes[33]	No[51]
Sterility[36,70]	Sterile if cut daily	Bacterial growth after 24 h of use
Side effects	Nil (as it is natural)	Fluoride poisoning cases reported due to fluoride toothpaste[75]
General body effects[20]	Yes	No

(1)

1.According to a study conducted in Saudi Arabia, Survival Rate of Oral Bacteria on Toothbrush and Miswak Stick were compared and it was found miswak significantly reduced the mean number of colony forming units during storage as compared with a toothbrush, thus the use of miswak after 24 hours can limit the risk for oral bacterial contamination and translocation.(3)

2. Both toothpaste and Miswak showed antibacterial effect against *S.aureus* and *C. albicans* in cold extracts and only Miwak hot aqueous extract indicated antimicrobial effect by modified agar well diffusion method and it was more effecient also Miwak is more efficient antifungal than antibacterial. For cultural growth before and after use of Miswak and toothpaste the table showed that using Miswak and toothpaste were effective in decreasing the microbial growth on nutrient agar plate but Miswak is more effective than toothpaste.(8)

3. It is thought that the increased secretion of thiocyanate and hydrogen peroxidase enzymes in the mouth enhances the germicidal systems in the saliva so that some harmful pathogens, especially *Aggregatibacter actinomycetemcomitans* were higher dominant in

the saliva of people who had used the industrial toothbrush rather than persica plant. In some studies, there were bacteria such as *A. actinomycetemcomitans, Staphylococcus intermedius, Veillonella parvula, Actinomyces israelii* and *Capnocytophaga gingivalis* bacteria and substantially in fewer amounts of *Selenomonas sputigena, Streptococcus salivarius, Streptococcus oralis* and *Actinomyces naeslundii* in the mouth of people who had used the toothbrush plant. Some other researches also reported a further reduction of *A. actinomycetemcomitans* when using industrial toothbrush compared to the use of toothbrush plant Hattab has considered more efficient the reduction of dental germs using the toothbrush plant rather than the industrial Oral-B toothbrush, and introduced both physical act and salivation caused by substances contained in plants persica the reason for the outcomes. In fact, physical cleansing is the first effective measure in brushing. Results showed that the antimicrobial properties of Miswak starts from the moment of entering the mouth and lasts a long time, while toothpaste has a very short durability so that is not comparable with Miswak(5)

4.Miswak has analgesic, astringent and anti-inflammatory properties, making it an effective treatment for primary periodontal diseases. it has been noted that patients practicing miswak regularly had a low incidence of toothache compared to toothbrush users.(1)

5.Numerous studies have identified that silica in miswak possesses plaque inhibiting properties, plays vital role in caries prevention and helps maintaining normal pH after acidogenic attacks chemically. The presence of calcium and chlorides in miswak inhibit the bacterial attachment on to the enamel surface hence providing a protective medium. In addition, miswak has an ability to remove plaque from the interproximal sites as well. This is due to better mechanical cleaning action of its fibers compared to fibers of conventional synthetic toothbrushes.(1)

6.Gazi et al reported that plaque and gingivitis were significantly reduced when miswak was used 5 times a day compared with conventional toothbrush. Guile et al concluded from a survey of Saudi school children that the low incidence of periodontal disease was attributable to the practice of using miswak for teeth cleaning.(9)

7. Almas and Al-Zeid tested the antimicrobial activity of Salvadora persica in vivo on Streptococcus mutans and Lactobacilli and found a marked reduction of Streptococcus mutans among all groups. When the groups were compared, the reduction of Streptoccus mutans was significantly greater using miswak in comparison to tooth brushing and there was no significant difference for Lactobacilli reduction.(9)

8. Several studies have shown that chewing stick is as or more effective than the toothbrush in reducing plaque and gingivitis by using the checkerboard hybridization technique to compare subgingival plaque samples of regular miswak and toothbrush users. Also Al-Khateeb et al. (1991) concluded that when miswak is used five times a day, it might offer a suitable alternative to a toothbrush for reducing plaque and gingivitis.(10)

9. A clinical trial study on Ethiopian school children comparing mefaka (Miswak) with conventional toothbrush, found Miswak to be as effective as the toothbrush in removing oral deposits. (6)

10. In a clinical trial among adolescents in Nigeria, the results showed that the *Massularia acuminata* chewing stick was as effective in controlling and removing dental plaque as the toothbrush and paste.(6)

11. Al-Otaibi et al., using the checkerboard DNA-DNA hybridization method, compared the effect of the miswak and a toothbrush on subgingival microbiota and reported a significantly greater reduction of subgingival A. actinomycetemcomitans by the miswak.(7)

12. A study was conducted to evaluate the efficacy of *Salvadora persica* (Miswak) products on cariogenic bacteria in comparison with ordinary toothpaste. Miswak mouthwash has a significant reduction effect on both bacteria immediately and after 2 weeks of use. Miswak toothpaste has a similar effect on Lactobacilli, while *Streptococcus mutans* showed a significant decrease only after 2 weeks of use in contrast to ordinary paste which showed a non significant effect on both bacteria at both time intervals .Hence Miswak products, especially mouth wash, were more effective in reducing the growth of cariogenic bacteria than ordinary toothpaste.(11)

13. In another study, there was significant immediate reduction in *streptococcus mutans* while comparing miswak with toothbrushing in salivary bacterial counts.(2, 12)

14. The results of a study on Miswak and toothpaste suggested that Miswak is more effective and safe antimicrobial toothbrush than toothpaste especialy that contain flouride. (8)

EPIDEMIOLOGICAL SURVEYS(effects on different oral health care parameters including caries, plaque and gingival scoring indices,pain and saliva secretion

1. The Consensus Statement on Oral Hygiene states that tooth brushing and other mechanical methods, including miswak ;chewing sticks are the most reliable means of controlling plaque, provided that the cleaning is sufficiently through and performed in regular base.(3)

2. According to a study conducted at muslim school in Lucknow ;oral hygiene status was assessed using the Gingival Index(1963), Oral Hygiene Index-Simplified (1964) and Plaque Index (1964). among miswaak users,toothbrush users and both muswaak and toothbrush users and was found Miswak users had lower mean gingival index score. Mean plaque score was lowest among combined users of toothbrush and miswak.(13)

3. According to another study conducted at Madharase Arabia Sirathe Mustakheem Bangalore city,plaque and gingival index were assessed between miswaak and tooth brush users and was found that miswaak was more effective in reducing plaque whereas both were equally effective in maintenance of gingival health.(14)

4.In a study conducted in Sudan,periodontal status of adult habitual miswak and toothbrush users was assessd. One examiner used the Community Periodontal Index (CPI) to score gingival bleeding, supragingival dental calculus, and probing pocket depth of the index teeth of each sextant. In addition, the attachment level was measured, which, along with the CPI, was used to assess the periodontal status of the two test groups.It was found that Miswak users had significantly lower dental calculus and probing depth and attachment loss as well as a tendency to lower gingival bleeding in the posterior sextants than did toothbrush users. These differences were not significant in the anterior sextants. (15)

5. Another study was conducted to compare the effect of the chewing stick (miswak), and toothbrushing on plaque removal and gingival health. Compared to tooth brushing, the use of the miswak resulted in significant reductions in plaque and gingival indices. (16)

6. Another study was done to compare the effectiveness of two oral hygiene aids: Chewing stick and manual toothbrush, for plaque removal and gingival health after one month of a randomized clinical trial and it was concluded that except for the mean plaque scores of toothbrush users (which increased at post-intervention examination), all other scores showed reduction. In contrast to the final mean gingival scores, a significant difference in the final mean plaque score was observed for the two respective interventional group. Chewing stick has revealed parallel and at times greater mechanical and chemical cleansing of oral tissues as compared to a toothbrush.(17)

7. The frequent use of miswak helps in reduction of plaque accumulation thus leading to a better oral hygiene. According to a study conducted in Kenya, miswak users (50 or over) had a very low incidence of periodontal diseases.Active miswak users reported better periodontal health, less gingival bleeding and interproximal bone loss compared to toothbrush users. Comparatively reduced gingival bleeding and low gingival indices score were observed in miswak users. Similar results were reported in a randomize control trials conducted by Al-Otaibi *et al*. A significant reduction in plaque score, gingival inflammation and bleeding of gums was observed in miswak users. Further, less tooth loss cases were reported in subjects who used miswak.(1)

8. Several studies have claimed that chewing sticks are effective in reducing plaque and gingival inflammation. (18)

 Results of another study using Gingival index according to Loe and Silness, Plaque index, according to Turesky modified Quigley-Hein plaque index, and the digital photographs of the total labial surfaces of the teeth showed significant improvement in plaque score and gingival health when miswak was used as an adjunct to tooth brushing. (18)

9. The results of another study conducted in India show that the subjects who were using both miswak as well as toothbrush and toothpaste were having better oral hygiene and had a lower plaque and gingival scores as scores as compared to the other groups either using only miswaak or only toothbrush for oral hygiene.(19)

10. Another study was done to check the effectiveness of natural toothbrush in pre-vention of dental caries and plaque formation. The plaque index and DMFT was assessed at the beginning of the study until 1 year. At the end of the study, the lowest plaque index was observed in the group using both the natural(miswaak) and artificial methods(tooth brushing and toothpaste). The increase in DMFT in the group that used artificial toothbrush was more than other groups using miswaak and both miswaak and toothbrush.Thus, use of natural toothbrush leads to a decrease in growth rate of DMFT.(20)

11. From another study, it was concluded that the study group using Miswak had less number of caries incidence than the control group of non-Miswaak users.(21)

12. Danielsen et al assessed the efficacy of brushing with chewing sticks on plaque removal and concludes that brushing with a chewing stick for five minutes resulted in a net reduction of the proportions of plaque deposit sites per child and the tooth paste resulted in no additional effect.(9)

13. Results of a study showed that miswak decoction injected intraperitoneally into mice, lower their response to chemical and thermal stimuli in the three analgesic tests. Miswak was more effective against thermal stimuli than against chemical stimuli. It is generally accepted that response to thermal stimuli is mediated via skin pain receptors while response to chemical stimuli is mediated via visceral receptors. Therefore, it was assumed that miswak is more effective against peripheral pain than visceral pain. This may explain the traditional claim that miswak decoction relieves oral pain by its application to oral mucosa.(6)

14. Sushil K. investigated the immediate and medium-term effect of Miswak on the composition of mixed saliva. Result of his study showed that chewing of miswak raised the level of calcium and chloride significantly when both the groups were pooled together. In a study conducted by Gazi et al.in1992 high amount of calcium and chloride were seen after chewing of miswak compared to corrugated rubber to stimulate salivery secreation. Thus it can be said that chewing miswaak has the potential to release such substances into saliva which can stimulate good oral health.(6)

15. The effects of aqueous extracts of chewing sticks (*Salvadora persica*) on the healthy and periodontally involved human dentine were evaluated with Scanning Electron Microscopy (SEM) *in vitro*. When the healthy and periodontally diseased root dentine was soaked in miswak extract it resulted in partial removal of smear layer and occlusion of tubules was observed in dentine specimens burnished with miswak solution. It was concluded that CHX 0.2% and miswak extract 50% had a similar effect on dentin in the control group. Miswak extract removed more smear layer as compared to CHX.(6)

DISADVANTAGES AND DAMAGES CAUSED BY TOOTHPASTE USE:

1.According to a study brushing habits of young children were observed and amount of fluoride retained and ingested after brushing with a fluoride toothpaste were evaluated and it was found that an average of 72% of the toothpaste applied to the brush was retained in the mouth and presumably ingested. The risk of **fluorosi**s is related to the dose of fluoride ingested and depends on both the amount of toothpaste ingested and its fluoride concentration. The permanent dentition is at risk of fluorosis during the first 7 years of life. Hence care must be taken to avoid risk of fluorosis.(22).

2.In a recent publication it says that as young infants and children under age 2 years can swallow most of the toothpaste when brushing, there has been concern that the use of fluoride toothpaste containing 1,000-1,500 ppm F could give rise to enamel fluorosis of the front permanent incisors. (8)

3.There are three published cases of fluoride toxicity associated with toothpaste ingestion.
a) The first case described skeletal fluorosis associated with toothpaste ingestion in a 45-year-old woman who complained of painful swelling of the fingers.(23)
b)The second case described a 52-year-old man who presented with osteosclerosis and elevated fluoride levels.(24)
c) In the third case a 58-year-old lady presented with a fracture in her foot.(25)
All these cases revealed large amount of fluoride ingestion through toothpaste.

(fluoride toothpaste –what are the dangers of chronic ingestion in adults?-------
Prepared by UK Medicines Information (UKMi) pharmacists for NHS healthcare professionals *Before using this Q&A, read the disclaimer at www.sps.nhs.uk/articles/about-ukmi-medicines-qas/*
Prepared: May 2014)

4.According to fluoride poisoning data collected by the American Association of Poison Control (AAPC),it was found that tooth paste ingestion remains the main source of toxicity followed by fluoride containing mouth washes and supplements. More than 80% of the cases of fluoride toxicity was reported in children below the age of 6 yrs. However, Chewing stick (miswak) is another option that is natural and there are no reports of fluoride toxicity from it's use.(26)

5. Toothpaste contains different potentially harmful ingredients some of which may lead to localized and systemic adverse effects. They have been mainly associated with fluoride, sodium lauryl sulphate (SLS), and triclosan. The local reaction includes oral mucosa irritation and desquamation (stomatitis, glossitis, gingivitis, buccal mucositis), while systemic ones are allergic and acute or chronic toxic reactions. According to the results of this study, fluorine dependent cytotoxic or genotoxic effect was not detected,whereas dentrifices with Sodium lauryl sulphate showed an increase in several cytogenetic parameters in buccal epithelial cells.(27)

6.NaF was found to decrease the cell viability of human gingival fibroblast in a dose- and timedependent manner .It also give rise to apoptotic morphological
changes including chromatin condensation, and DNA fragmentation,which demonstrates that fluoride induces apoptosis in human gingival fibroblasts.(28)

7.According to a study, under in vivo conditions, the acute topical appliance of fluoride gel (NaF 2%) on teeth was shown to induce a significant level of DNA damage/genotoxic effect in the oral epithelial cells.(29)

8.Studies show that SLS-containing toothpaste is associated with a more frequent occurrence of inflammation and desquamation of oral mucosa.(30, 31)
Siegel and Gordon found that SLS, even at low concentrations, was found to reduce the protective barrier function of the oral epithelium. Widening of the stratum corneum, due to separation and loss of surface epithelial layers.(31)

9.According to a case report a patient presented with sore throat and fever.Upon observation Aphthous ulcer of the uvula was seen.His symptoms exacerbated with burping .The patient had history of recurrent aphthous stomatitis but last relapse has been several years ago.He realized that he had accidentally been using a toothpaste containing sodium lauryl sulfate for a few weeks prior to symptom onset. He has not experienced any recurrences upon switching back to his regular toothpaste without sodium lauryl sulfate.This again shows harmful effects of such toothpaste on oral mucosal health.(32)

10.The minimal risk level for daily oral fluoride uptake was determined to be 0.05 mg/kg/day which was based on a non-observable adverse effect level (NOAEL) of 0.15mgfluoride/kg/day for an increased fracture rate. Estimations of human lethal fluoride doses showed a wide range of values, from 16 to 64 mg/kg in adults and 3 to
 16 mg/kg in children.
Fluoride exerts diverse cellular effects in a time-, concentration-, and cell-type-dependent manner. The main toxic effect of fluoride in cells consists of its interaction with enzymes. Research data strongly suggest that fluoride inhibits protein secretion and/or synthesis and that it influences distinct signaling pathways involved in proliferation and apoptosis.
The cytotoxic effects of fluoride occur in all cell types. However, time and concentration-dependent responses are different from one cell type to another. Necrosis has been observed as a primary mechanism of cell death in the presence of relatively high fluoride concentrations.
Fluoride induces apoptosis by elevating oxidative stress-induced lipid peroxidation, thus causing mitochondrial dysfunction and the activation of downstream pathways.
Many works have reported the role of intracellular calcium content in fluoride-induced apoptosis as a direct target of toxicity or an indirect consequence of altered cellular processes.Another component of apoptotic signaling is the expression/regulation of pro- and anti-apoptotic genes. For example, Bcl-2 has been demonstrated to be involved in fluoride-induced apoptosis.In the presence of 20mMNaF, human gingival fibroblasts (HGF cells) showed a down-regulation of Bcl-2 followed by the activation of amitochondrial cell death pathway.
Thus, concentrations of 5–7.5mM NaF are capable of inducing Apoptosis.

Dental fluorosis is a clear case in point of fluoride's influence on secretory pathways. It was quickly established that either acute or chronic exposure to NaF affects enamel formation, triggering dental fluorosis that manifests as mottled, discolored and porous enamel. Aoba and Fejerskov suggested that these effects areassociated with precipitation of by fluoride ions,altering enamel mineralization. Alternatively, several authors concluded that these clinical signs are associated with the action of fluoride on the secretory functions of ameloblasts, epithelial cells responsible for enamel development.(33) The biological mechanism was recently elucidated and involves the ER stress response resulting in a reduction of protein synthesis, secretion and total protein concentration.

11. Fluoride could influence the transcription pattern without inducing cell stress or apoptosis. In odontoblasts in vivo, aberrant expression of these fluoride-sensitive genes may impair the formation of the extracellular matrix and influence cell communication, with the possible consequence of fluorotic patterns of normal and deviant dentin.(34)

12. According to a study the no. of cases reported for fluoride toxicity have been increased in 1985 and 1986. About two percent of the reports involved "adult vitamin" products;37% involved "pediatric vitamins"; **61%** involved sources of fluoride other than vitamins. As they are the most widely available sources of large quantities of fluoride, the latter group would be largely represented by dental products for home use- products such as dentifrices, mouthrinses, and supplemental tablets. Thus, it may be concluded that the over-ingestion of these products occurs on casual basis.(35)
Based on reports, it is concluded that the PTD(probably toxic dose)of fluoride is approximately 5 mg F/kg.The above considerations indicate that the quantities of fluoride contained in some dental products exceed the PTD for small children. For example, the PTD for a 2-year-old child of average body weight (11.3 kg) is 57 mg. This quantity is contained in 57 g (2 ounces) of a 1000-ppm-f1uoride dentifrice,38 g of a 1500-ppm dentifrice, 248 mL of a 0.05% sodium fluoride mouthrinse, 57 1.0-mg fluoride tablets, and only 4.6 mL of a 1.23% APF gel. With the exception of the tablets,these products have a long history of use without a report of serious acute toxicity. Nevertheless, it is clear that a hazard still exists.
There are, several published reports which indicate that daily fluoride ingestion associated with the use of topical fluoride products can easily equal or exceed the intake from dietary sources, even in communities where the water fluoride level is considered optimal (Hellstrom,1960; Ericsson and Forsman, 1969; Hargreaves et al.,1972; Parkins, 1972; Barnhart et al., 1974; Aasenden and Peebles, 1974; Baxter, 1980; Dowell, 1981; Wei and Kanellis,1983; Bell et al., 1985; Whitford et al., 1987; Larsen et al.,1987; Bruun and Thylstrup, 1988). Based on these reports, we can consider that by the age of 18 months, approximately 75% of the children brush or have their teeth brushed with a fluoride containing dentifrice. The average quantity of dentifrice or mouth rinse involved per use contains 1.0 mg of fluoride, although the range is from 0.1 to over 3.0 mg; that, of the fluoride which is introduced into the mouth with each use of a dentifrice or mouthrinse, an average of about 25-30% is ingested and the range of ingested fluoride is from less than ten percent to nearly 100%, and the fraction swallowed is inversely proportional to age, which indicates younger children ingest more. Therefore, an unintended fluoride "supplement" is taken with each use of dentifrice, mouth rinse, or any other product designed for topical application, regardless of the fluoride concentrations of drinking water or other dietary

components. In view of the small difference(ca 0.25 mg per day in an optimally fluoridated area;ca.0.4mg per day where the drinking water fluoride level is less but 0.3 ppm higher) between the level of daily fluoride intake considered optimal for caries control
and the level associated with an unacceptable degree of dental fluorosis, it would be very surprising if the prevalence of dental fluorosis had not increased. They also urge strict adherence to the current guidelines for the prescription of dietary fluoride supplements.(35)

13. Previously done studies have demonstrated that toothpastes contain a number of ingredients that can remove not only the oral biofilm but also the superficial dentin tissue. Among these components, abrasives and detergents are most common. In this study also the main component associated with the adverse effects of the toothpastes was more likely to be the sodium lauryl sulphate because this anionic detergent can cause adverse effects on cells, as a consequence of its ionic properties, responsible for initiating the process of cell death. Only the toothpates containing probably lower concentration of this detergent proved to be biocompatible. Another component that has been associated with the cytotoxicity of oral mucosa is **triclosan,**an active ingredient used in toothpastes, which presents antibacterial activity and an anti-plaque effect however ,toothpaste containing combination of triclosan and NaF produced highly cytotoxic effects. (36)

14.Detergents have also been found to be involved in the abrasive potential of toothpastes. In a study by Moore and Addy it was showed that detergents can modulate the effect of abrasives in dentin wear in a way that may reflect the rheological properties of the mixture. According to these authors, **sodium lauryl sulphate** class of detergents is the most aggressive in terms of abrasiveness.(37)

15. Neppelberg *et al* also have already shown a direct correlation between sodium lauryl sulphate concentration and cell death in epithelial cells in his study.(38)

16.An in vitro study that evaluated the toxicology of triclosan at the cellular level showed that this ingredient damages the integrity of the plasma membrane, and apparently induces cell death by apoptosis. Moreover, these authors observed that the combination of triclosan with NaF or Zn citrate increased the cytotoxic potential of the triclosan.(39)

17.In a study on patients with recurrent aphthous ulcers it was found that a significantly higher number of ulcers were seen in patients brushing with sodium lauryl sulphate containing toothpastes.(40)

18. Based on the risks and benefits of fluoride toothpaste use by young Australian children it was seen that the use of a high amount of toothpaste and the habit of swallowing or licking the toothpaste resulted in an increased risk of fluorosis, without a significant improvement in anticaries effect .(41)

19.The toothpastes tested in the study had some degree of toxicity and their cytotoxity appeared to be increased significantly causing cell death with an increase in the time of exposure.

> The research conducted by Gerckens and Herlofson also revealed that SLS is the most toxic agent on mucosal cells and causes epithelial desquamation.
> Other ingredients including sodium monofluorophosphate, silicone dioxide, hydrated silica, sodium benzoate, preservatives, colors, flavors, and essences may also produce toxic and harmful effects.(42)

20.Whitening toothpastes have been found to be more cytotoxic as well as genotoxic to the cells in vitro than the common toothpastes.(43)

21. Toothpaste ingredients may become harmful if ingested, particularly by children or people with learning disability, and may contribute to damage to hard tissues (abrasion, staining)of teeth and occasionally soft-tissues like oral mucosa.
> Fluoride may be ingested from toothpaste by young children can result in fluorosis . The risk of fluorosis is related to the dose of fluoride ingested that means the fluoride concentration x amount. The amount of toothpaste poses a greater risk than the fluoride concentration(44). Toothpaste alone was responsible for an average of 81.5% of the daily fluoride intake in pre-school Brazilian children.(45)
> Sodium lauryl sulphate (SLS) is a detergent commonly used in toothpaste and may occasionally cause mucosal desquamation or ulceration.
> In 2005, a "toothpaste cancer alert" appeared after a report that triclosan can react with water to produce chloroform which, if inhaled in large amounts can cause depression, liver problems and, in some cases, cancer.
> Soft tissue reactions may also occur, most often to essential oils, flavourings, cinnamonaldehyde, benzoates, or carvone, and manifest as direct irritants or allergic reactions in the mouth, lips as contact cheilitis. Rarely allergic rhinitis or asthma may occur. Essential oils, such as peppermint, anethole, cinnamon, cloves and spearmint and antimicrobial agents can cause cheilitis or circumoral dermatitis. Carvone is a common constituent of essential oils and may be implicated. Some toothpaste ingredients have been implicated in other reactions. Tartar-control pyrophosphate dentifrices occasionally cause erythema, scaling and fissuring of the perioral area, sometimes with cheilitis, gingivitis and circumoral dermatitis and other reactions. (44)

22.According to another study tartar control toothpastes resulted in statistically significant rates of mucosal reactions (e.g., ulceration, sloughing, erythema, migratory glossitis) than the non-tartar control toothpastes .(46)

23.

COMPARISON OF FRESH AND OLD MISWAAK EFFECTS ON ORAL HEALTH AND INDEX SCORES

✓ According to study, fresh miswaak soaked in water for 24 hours is preferred for use.Moreover,the presence of odourous components is considered good indicator for tooth brushing efficiency.The same head is not recommended for use after 24 hours because of cytotoxic activity.In this study the hot extract was less in its antimicrobial effect than the cold one this is may be due to loss of some active ingredients by hot water. So it is recommended to use fresh Miswak and if soaked in cold not hot water before use.(8)

✓ It has been demonstrated that freshly cut miswak has no cytotoxic effect on oral health. But same miswak used after 24 h contained toxins harmful for the oral and general health.(1)Thus once after use,another brush is made from the rest of the stick.That's why it is recommended to renew the head of the miswaak and use a fresh head as often as possible.The optimal way is to use the crushed part until it loses it's taste and odour.At that point the overused end has to be cut off because of the presence of odorous components is considered a good indicator for tooth brush efficiency.(10)

✓ According to a study conducted in Sweden fresh roots of S.persica were taken from Saudia Arabia and analyzed experimentally. The main anti bacterial compound in *S.persica* essential oil was found to be benzyl isothiocyanate (BICT) released from the Miswak chewing sticks into the saliva during use.The study results also show that the amount of BITC released from the Miswak reduced drastically if the same Miswak is used more than once.The findings suggest that in order to achieve any chemical effect besides the mechanical it would be necessary to use a fresh piece of Miswak each time. Thus it is recommended to regularly change/cut the tip of the Miswak in order to optimize its effect.(47)

COMPARISON BETWEEN DIFFERENT TYPES OF MISWAAK AND DIFFERENCES IN THEIR EFFECTS ,CHEMICAL COMPOSITION AND ANTIMICROBIAL ACTIVITY

Types of miswaak:

Table 1: Different types of chewing sticks

S. No.	Plants	Local name	Parts used	Useful properties
1	Salvodora persica	Miswak	Fresh young part of stem /branches	Astringent, antibacterial
2	Azadirachta indica (meliaceal)	Neem	Stem, branches	Bitter, astringent, antiseptic, antibacterial, analgesic, anti-inflammatory, antiviral, antifungal.
3	Acacia Catechu (Mimosaceae)	Khair	Stem, bark	Astringent, cooling, antiseptic, anti-inflammatory, bitter.
4	Acacia nilotica (Mimosaceae)	Kikar	Stem, branches	Astringent, styptic, antibacterial, antifungal, acrid.
5	Acacia leucophloea (Mimosaceae)	Safed babul	Stem, branches	Astringent, styptic, antibacterial, antifungal.
6	Achyranthes aspera (Amaranthaceal)	Apamarga	Stem, bark	Anti-inflammatory.
7	Aegle marmelos (Rutaceae)	Bael tree	Stem, branches	Astringent, antibacterial.
8	Butea monosperma (fabaceae)	Dhak	Stem, branches	Astringent, bitter, antibacterial, anti-inflammatory, antifungal.
9	Calotropis procera/ (Asclepiadaceae)	Madar, AK	Stem	Astringent, antimicrobial, antiseptic, styptic.
10	Nerium indicum	Kamer	Stem, branches	Antibacterial, analgesic, anti-inflammatory, antifungal.
11	Pongamia pinnata (fabaceae)	Karanj	Stem, root	Astringent, styptic, antiseptic, antibacterial, antifungal.
12	Pterocarpus marsupium (fabaceae)	Vijayasar	Stem	Astringent, styptic, antifungal, anti-inflammatory.
13	Terminalia arjuna (conufretaceae)	Arjun	Stem, branches	Astringent, styptic, cooling, demulcent, antibacterial, antifungal.
14	Ficus racemosa (Moraceae)	Gular	Stem, branches and bark	Astringent, antiseptic, antifungal, anti-inflammatory.
15	Ficus fenghalensis (Moraceae)	Bargad	Stem, branches	Astringent, styptic, anti-inflammatory, analgesic, antioxidant.
16	Glycyrrhiza glabra (fabaceae)	Mulhatti	Stem, branches	Demulcent, haemostatic, antimicrobial, anti-inflammatory, antiviral, analgesic.
17	Zanthoxylum aromatum	Tejovati	Stem, branches	Astringent, antiseptic, antibacterial.

- Commonly practiced species are *S. persica* (Peelu), *Azadirachta indica* (Neem), *Olea europaea* (Zaitoon), *Acacia arabica* (Kikar), *Glycosmis pentaphylla* (Ban), *Capparis aphylla* (Khiran).Most of these sticks are easily available in different parts of Pakistan, Middle East and African countries. Arak (*S. persica*) is the most commonly used miswak in Saudi Arabia while litmus and orange tree are common in West Africa.*S. persica* obtained from Arak tree is the most popular having spongy characteristics and stem that can easily be crushed between teeth. (1)

- The total fluoride content of Miswak sticks is ap-proximately 1.02 µg/g. Farah realized that SP chewable sticks, Neem-kikar, walnut and Pekujebu con-tain 2.8, 1.0, 0.5 and 0.2 µg/ml fluoride, respectively. Crystallographic assessment with fluorescence and mi-croanalysis with X ray showed that *Salvadora persica* contains more calcium and phosphorous.(20)Also a study by Chawla reported that some types of chewing sticks such as Neem *(Azadirachta indica),Salvadora persica* and *Acacia arabica* contain a reasonable amount of fluoride.(6)

- According to a study conducted at Riyadh,samples of the most commonly used chewing sticks in Pakistan Neem (Azadirechta Indica), Zaitoon (Olea europaea),Kikar (Accacia arabica), Peelu (Salvadora persica), Ban (Glycosmic pentaphylla), Khiran (Capparis aphylla) and Arak (Salvadora persica) from Saudi Arabia were bought from the open market and their antimicrobial effects were compared. It was found that there was no antimicrobial effect at low concentration of chewing sticks extracts but was found on Streptococcus fecalis at 50% concentration of kikar(Acacia arabia) from Pakistan and Arak (Salvadora persica)from Saudi Arabia. The inhibition zones up to 2 mm were found in these two chewing sticks extracts.(48)

- According to a study conducted in India,the anti microbial efficacy of four chewing sticks including neem,miswaak(salvadora persica),mango and banyan was compared and was found that neem aqueous extracts showed the the most anti microbial activity against Streptococcus mutans whereas miswaak extracts showed against Lactobacillus acidophilus and their activity was directly proportional to the concentration of the extracts.Although banyan extracts showed no anti microbial activity yet widely used due to it's good mechanical properties.(49)

- According to another study four different types of miswaks i.e. (1) rootof the peelu (*Salvadora persica)* tree (in packing) (2) root of the peelu tree (without packing) (3) stem of the peelu tree & (4) stem of the neem (*Azadirechta indica)* tree were taken and their anti microbial activity was tested against three different types of microorganisms isolated from oral swabs: *Staphylococcus aureus, Streptococcus mutans* & *Candida albicans.It was found that* root of the peelu tree in both packing and without packing exhibited strong antimicrobial effect against all three tested microorganisms. However miswak taken from the stem of the peelu and neem tree did not show any antimicrobial activity against all three types of the tested microorganisms.(50)

KEY POINTS

❖ Various biological components present in miswaak are known to produce beneficial effects on oral health.It causes increased saliva production and through certain anti microbial agents and chemicals has effective role in prevention of oral diseases and infections including plaque,gingivitis,periodontitis and caries.

❖ Upon comparing survival rate of oral bacteria on toothbrush and miswaak stick after 24hrs of use,it was found that total oral bacterial survival rate was significantly reduced in miswaak users in comparison to toothbrush users.

❖ Fluoride poisoning cases are also reported due to swallowing of fluoride toothpastes.

❖ Numerous studies prove miswaak to be more efficient in reducing plaque,gingival,periodontal and caries indices in comparison to the use of toothbrush and toothpaste owing to its natural antimicrobial,mechanical and chemical properties.

❖ Fresh miswaak soaked in fresh water for 24hrs is preferred for use.The same head is not recommended for use after 24 hrs because of developing cytotoxic activity and harmful effects.The amount of main antimicrobial agent; benzyl isothiocyanate in Salvadora persica is found to reduce drastically after 24hrs.Hence head of miswaak should be renewed as often as possible.

❖ The most commonly practised miswak comes from peelu,neem,zaitoon,kikar,ban and khiran.

❖ Salvadora persica miswaak contains more total floride content as compared to other few miswaaks.It also contains more calcium and phosphorous.

❖ Different studies show variations in anti microbial efficacy of chewing sticks upon testing against different types of microorganisms.

REFERENCES:

1.   Niazi F, Naseem M, Khurshid Z, Zafar MS, Almas K. Role of Salvadora persica chewing stick (miswak): A natural toothbrush for holistic oral health. European Journal of Dentistry. 2016;10(2):301-8.
2.   Sukkarwalla A, Ali SM, Lundberg P, Tanwir F. Efficacy of miswak on oral pathogens. Dental research journal. 2013;10(3):314.
3.   Darout IA, Homeida HE. Survival Rate of Oral Bacteria on Toothbrush and Miswak Stick. American Journal of Health Research. 2016;4(5):134-7.
4.   Sofrata AH. Salvadora persica (MISWAK): An effective way of killing oral pathogens: Institutionen för odontologi/Department of Odontology; 2010.
5.   Biglari H, Saeidi M, Sohrabi Y, Khaksefidi R, Rahdar S, Narooie M, et al. Persica a miracle in the protect and promote oral and dental health. International Journal of Pharmacy and Technology. 2016;8(3):17957-67.
6.   Dutta S, Shaikh A. The active chemical constituent and biological activity of Salvadora persica (Miswak).
7.   Sofrata AH, Claesson RL, Lingström PK, Gustafsson AK. Strong antibacterial effect of miswak against oral microorganisms associated with periodontitis and caries. Journal of periodontology. 2008;79(8):1474-9.
8.   El-Desoukey RM. Comparative microbiological study between the Miswak (Salvadora persica) and the toothpaste. 2015.
9.   Hooda A, Rathee M, Singh J. Chewing Sticks In The Era Of Toothbrush A Review2009.
10.   Ahmad H, Ahamed N. Therapeutic properties of meswak chewing sticks: A review. African Journal of Biotechnology. 2012;11(83):14850-7.
11.   Al-Dabbagh SA, Qasim HJ, Al-Derzi NA. Efficacy of Miswak toothpaste and mouthwash on cariogenic bacteria. Saudi Medical Journal. 2016;37(9):1009-14.
12.   Almas K, Al-Zeid Z. The immediate antimicrobial effect of a toothbrush and miswak on cariogenic bacteria: a clinical study. The journal of contemporary dental practice. 2004;5(1):105-14.
13.   Saha S, Mohammad S, Saha S, Samadi F. Efficiency of traditional chewing stick (miswak) as an oral hygiene aid among Muslim school children in Lucknow: A cross-sectional study. Journal of oral biology and craniofacial research. 2012;2(3):176-80.
14.   Shankar S. Evaluation of comparative effect of chewing stick (miswak) and manual toothbrush on plaque removal and maintenance of gingival health: RGUHS; 2008.
15.   Darout IA, Albandar JM, Skaug N. Periodontal status of adult Sudanese habitual users of miswak chewing sticks or toothbrushes. Acta Odontologica Scandinavica. 2000;58(1):25-30.
16.   Al-Otaibi M, Al-Harthy M, Soder B, Gustafsson A, Angmar-Mansson B. Comparative effect of chewing sticks and toothbrushing on plaque removal and gingival health. Oral health & preventive dentistry. 2003;1(4):301-7.
17.   Malik AS, Shaukat MS, Qureshi AA, Abdur R. Comparative Effectiveness of Chewing Stick and Toothbrush: A Randomized Clinical Trial. North American Journal of Medical Sciences. 2014;6(7):333-7.
18.   Patel PV, Shruthi S, Kumar S. Clinical effect of miswak as an adjunct to tooth brushing on gingivitis. Journal of Indian Society of Periodontology. 2012;16(1):84.

19. Shah AF, Yousuf A, Sidiq M, Baba IA, Jan SM. Comparative Evaluation of Conventional Toothbrushing with Traditional Miswak for Oral Hygiene Maintainence in a Socially Disadvantaged Young Muslim Population.

20. Ezoddini-Ardakani M, Shadkam MN, Fotouhi H, Kashani FB, Abbassi M, Hashemian Z, et al. Study of the effects of natural toothbrush (Salvadora persica) in prevention of dental caries and plaque index. 2012.

21. Al Jeaidi Z, Mustafa M. Study of caries prevalence among miswak and non-miswak users: a prospective study. Dent Pract. 2016;17(11):926-9.

22. Bentley EM, Ellwood RP, Davies RM. Fluoride ingestion from toothpaste by young children. Br Dent J. 1999;186(9):460-2.

23. Roos J, Dumolard A, Bourget S, Grange L, Rousseau A, Gaudin P, et al. [Osteofluorosis caused by excess use of toothpaste]. Presse medicale (Paris, France : 1983). 2005;34(20 Pt 1):1518-20.

24. Kurland ES, Schulman RC, Zerwekh JE, Reinus WR, Dempster DW, Whyte MP. Recovery from skeletal fluorosis (an enigmatic, American case). Journal of bone and mineral research : the official journal of the American Society for Bone and Mineral Research. 2007;22(1):163-70.

25. Joshi S, Hlaing T, Whitford GM, Compston JE. Skeletal fluorosis due to excessive tea and toothpaste consumption. Osteoporosis international : a journal established as result of cooperation between the European Foundation for Osteoporosis and the National Osteoporosis Foundation of the USA. 2011;22(9):2557-60.

26. Ullah R, Zafar MS, Shahani N. Potential fluoride toxicity from oral medicaments: A review. Iranian journal of basic medical sciences. 2017;20(8):841.

27. Tadin A, Gavic L, Govic T, Galic N, Zorica Vladislavic N, Zeljezic D. In vivo evaluation of fluoride and sodium lauryl sulphate in toothpaste on buccal epithelial cells toxicity. Acta Odontologica Scandinavica. 2019;77(5):386-93.

28. Lee JH, Jung JY, Jeong YJ, Park JH, Yang KH, Choi NK, et al. Involvement of both mitochondrial- and death receptor-dependent apoptotic pathways regulated by Bcl-2 family in sodium fluoride-induced apoptosis of the human gingival fibroblasts. Toxicology. 2008;243(3):340-7.

29. VAZQUEZ-ALVARADOsup P, MELENDEZ-OCAMPO A, ORTIZ-ESPINOSA RM, MUNtilde S. Genotoxic damage in oral epithelial cells induced by fluoride in drinking-water on students of Tula de Allende, Hidalgo, Mexico. Journal of Toxicology and Environmental Health Sciences. 2012;4(8):123-9.

30. Herlofson BB, Barkvoll P. Desquamative effect of sodium lauryl sulfate on oral mucosa. A preliminary study. Acta Odontol Scand. 1993;51(1):39-43.

31. Herlofson BB, Barkvoll P. Oral mucosal desquamation caused by two toothpaste detergents in an experimental model. European journal of oral sciences. 1996;104(1):21-6.

32. Pareek M, Bhatt DL. The Wrong Toothpaste and the Painful Burp. The American Journal of Medicine. 2017;130(1):e19-e20.

33. Barbier O, Arreola-Mendoza L, Del Razo LM. Molecular mechanisms of fluoride toxicity. Chemico-biological interactions. 2010;188(2):319-33.

34. Wurtz T, Houari S, Mauro N, MacDougall M, Peters H, Berdal A. Fluoride at non-toxic dose affects odontoblast gene expression in vitro. Toxicology. 2008;249(1):26-34.

35. Whitford GM. The physiological and toxicological characteristics of fluoride. Journal of Dental Research. 1990;69(2_suppl):539-49.

36.   SOUZA-RODRIGUES RD, FERREIRA SdS, D ALMEIDA-COUTO RS, LACHOWSKI KM, SOBRAL MÂP, MARQUES MM. Choice of toothpaste for the elderly: an in vitro study. Brazilian Oral Research. 2015;29:1-7.

37.   Moore C, Addy M. Wear of dentine in vitro by toothpaste abrasives and detergents alone and combined. Journal of clinical periodontology. 2005;32(12):1242-6.

38.   Neppelberg E, Costea DE, Vintermyr OK, Johannessen AC. Dual effects of sodium lauryl sulphate on human oral epithelial structure. Experimental dermatology. 2007;16(7):574-9.

39.   Zuckerbraun HL, Babich H, May R, Sinensky MC. Triclosan: cytotoxicity, mode of action, and induction of apoptosis in human gingival cells in vitro. European journal of oral sciences. 1998;106(2 Pt 1):628.

40.   Herlofson BB, Barkvoll P. The effect of two toothpaste detergents on the frequency of recurrent aphthous ulcers. Acta Odontol Scand. 1996;54(3):150-3.

41.   Do LG, Spencer AJ. Risk-benefit balance in the use of fluoride among young children. J Dent Res. 2007;86(8):723-8.

42.   Ghapanchi J, Kamali F, Moattari A, Poorshahidi S, Shahin E, Rezazadeh F, et al. In vitro comparison of cytotoxic and antibacterial effects of 16 commercial toothpastes. Journal of international oral health: JIOH. 2015;7(3):39.

43.   Camargo SE, Jóias RP, Santana-Melo GF, Ferreira LT, El Achkar VN, Rode Sde M. Conventional and whitening toothpastes: cytotoxicity, genotoxicity and effect on the enamel surface. Am J Dent. 2014;27(6):307-11.

44.   Davies R, Scully C, Preston AJ. Dentifrices-an update. Med Oral Patol Oral Cir Bucal. 2010;15(6):e976-82.

45.   de Almeida BS, da Silva Cardoso VE, Buzalaf MA. Fluoride ingestion from toothpaste and diet in 1- to 3-year-old Brazilian children. Community dentistry and oral epidemiology. 2007;35(1):53-63.

46.   Kowitz G, Jacobson J, Meng Z, Lucatorto F. The effects of tartar-control toothpaste on the oral soft tissues. Oral surgery, oral medicine, and oral pathology. 1990;70(4):529-36.

47.   Albabtain R, Azeem M, Wondimu Z, Lindberg T, Borg-Karlson AK, Gustafsson A. Investigations of a Possible Chemical Effect of Salvadora persica Chewing Sticks. Evidence-Based Complementary and Alternative Medicine. 2017;2017.

48.   Almas K. The antimicrobial effects of seven different types of Asian chewing sticks.

49.   Elangovan A, Muranga J, Joseph E. Comparative evaluation of the antimicrobial efficacy of four chewing sticks commonly used in South India: An in vitro study. Indian Journal of Dental Research. 2012;23(6):840.

50.   Naseem S, Hashmi K, Fasih F, Sharafat S, Khanani R. In vitro evaluation of antimicrobial effect of miswak against common oral pathogens. Pakistan journal of medical sciences. 2014;30(2):398.

YOUR KNOWLEDGE HAS VALUE

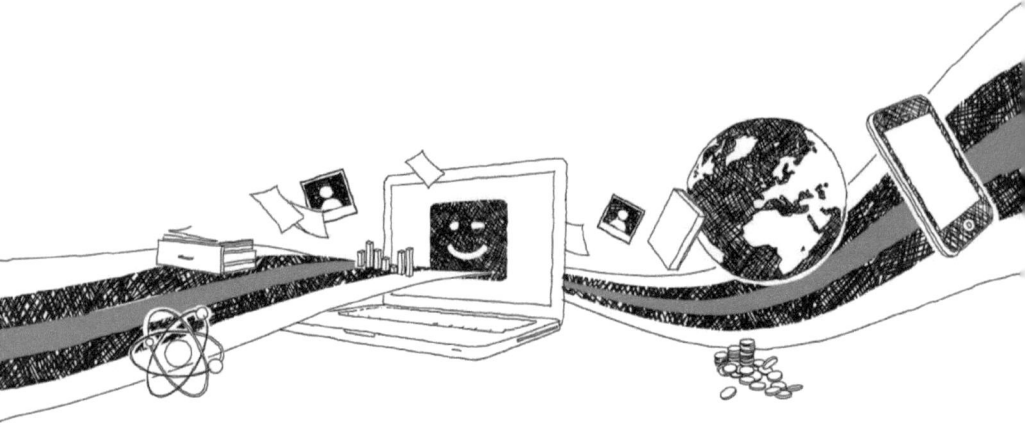

- We will publish your bachelor's and
  master's thesis, essays and papers

- Your own eBook and book -
  sold worldwide in all relevant shops

- Earn money with each sale

Upload your text at www.GRIN.com
and publish for free

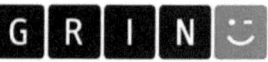